From the Institute o
National Research Council Report

MW00910532

Confronting Commercial Sexual Exploitation

and

Sex Trafficking of Minors

in the United States

A Guide for the Health Care Sector

INSTITUTE OF MEDICINE *AND*
NATIONAL RESEARCH COUNCIL
OF THE NATIONAL ACADEMIES

In 2013, the Institute of Medicine (IOM) and the National Research Council (NRC) published a report about commercial sexual exploitation and sex trafficking of minors in the United States. The report, *Confronting Commercial Sexual Exploitation and Sex Trafficking of Minors in the United States*, was funded by the U.S. Department of Justice Office of Juvenile Justice and Delinquency Prevention. It provides a comprehensive view of this issue and offers a detailed explanation of its findings and recommendations.

The content of this guide was derived entirely from the original report as an abridged version for professionals in the health care sector. This guide, which was also funded by the U.S. Department of Justice Office of Juvenile Justice and Delinquency Prevention, was edited by Rona Briere and Patti Simon.

Confronting Commercial Sexual Exploitation and Sex Trafficking of Minors in the United States was authored by the IOM/NRC Committee on the Commercial Sexual Exploitation and Sex Trafficking of Minors in the United States:

ELLEN WRIGHT CLAYTON (*Co-Chair*), Craig-Weaver Professor of Pediatrics, Professor of Law, and Co-Founder, Center for Biomedical Ethics and Society, Vanderbilt University

RICHARD D. KRUGMAN (*Co-Chair*), Vice Chancellor for Health Affairs, University of Colorado School of Medicine

TONYA CHAFFEE, Medical Director of Child and Adolescent Support, Advocacy and Resource Center, University of California, San Francisco

ANGELA DIAZ, Jean C. and James W. Crystal Professor of Pediatrics and Preventive Medicine, Mount Sinai School of Medicine

ABIGAIL ENGLISH, Director, Center for Adolescent Health & the Law

BARBARA GUTHRIE, Associate Dean for Academic Affairs and Professor, Yale University School of Nursing

SHARON LAMBERT, Associate Professor of Clinical/Community Psychology, The George Washington University

MARK LATONERO, Research Director, Annenberg Center on Communication Leadership & Policy, University of Southern California

NATALIE McCLAIN, Assistant Professor, Boston College William F. Connell School of Nursing

CALLIE MARIE RENNISON, Associate Professor, School of Public Affairs, University of Colorado Denver

JOHN A. RICH, Professor and Chair of Health Management and Policy, Drexel University School of Public Health

JONATHAN TODRES, Professor of Law, Georgia State University College of Law

PATTI TOTH, Program Manager, Washington State Criminal Justice Training Commission

International Standard Book Number-13: 978-0-309-31043-7
International Standard Book Number-10: 0-309-31043-1

Additional copies of this report are available from the National Academies Press, 500 Fifth Street, NW, Keck 360, Washington, DC 20001; (800) 624-6242 or (202) 334-3313; http://www.nap.edu.

Contents

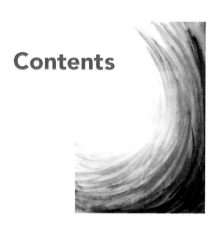

1 Introduction

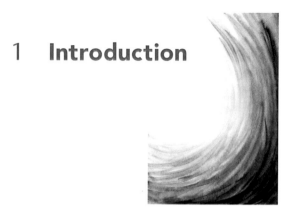

"Commercial sexual exploitation and sex trafficking of minors not only are illegal activities, but also result in immediate and long-term physical, mental, and emotional harm to victims and survivors."

Commercial sexual exploitation and sex trafficking of minors in the United States are frequently overlooked, misunderstood, and unaddressed domestic problems. In the past decade, they have received increasing attention from advocates, the media, academics, and policy makers. However, much of this attention has focused internationally. This international focus has overshadowed the reality that commercial sexual exploitation and sex trafficking of minors also occur every day within the United States.

Commercial sexual exploitation and sex trafficking of minors not only are illegal activities, but also result in immediate and long-term physical, mental, and emotional harm to victims and survivors. A nation that is unaware of these problems or disengaged from solving them unwittingly contributes to the ongoing abuse of minors and all but ensures that these crimes will remain marginalized and misunderstood.

PURPOSE OF THIS GUIDE

In September 2013, the Institute of Medicine (IOM) and the National Research Council (NRC) of the National Academies published the report *Confronting*

Commercial Sexual Exploitation and Sex Trafficking of Minors in the United States
[1]. The purpose of that report is

- to increase awareness and understanding of the crucial problem of commercial sexual exploitation and sex trafficking of minors in the United States;
- to examine emerging strategies for preventing and identifying these crimes, for assisting and supporting victims and survivors, and for addressing exploiters and traffickers; and
- to offer a path forward through recommendations designed to increase awareness and understanding and to support efforts to prevent, identify, and respond to these crimes.

The IOM/NRC report includes chapters on specific sectors with a role to play in addressing the problem. Because the report is lengthy and broad in its reach, the IOM/NRC, with the support of the U.S. Department of Justice Office of Juvenile Justice and Delinquency Prevention, decided to develop a series of guides offering a more concise and focused perspective on the problem and emerging solutions for several of these sectors.

INTENDED AUDIENCE

The intended audience for this guide is health care professionals, such as physicians, nurses, advanced practice nurses, physician assistants, mental health professionals, and dentists, who see children and adolescents for prevention and treatment of injury, illness, and disease. At any of these encounters—in settings that include, among others, emergency departments, urgent care, primary care clinics, adolescent medicine clinics, school clinics, shelters, specialty clinics (obstetrics/gynecology, psychiatry), community health centers, health department clinics, free-standing Title X clinics, Planned Parenthood, and dental clinics [2]—these health care professionals can have an opportunity to identify and assist young people who are victims of commercial sexual exploitation and sex trafficking [3, 4, 5, 6, 7, 8].

Ideally, these professionals would be involved in efforts focused on the prevention of victimization by these crimes and work to identify and provide treatment/referral for victims and survivors. Yet despite the potential opportunities for intervention, health care professionals often overlook or fail to identify these youth. The result can be missed opportunities for intervention and the continued perpetration of these crimes. This guide is intended to raise awareness of these opportunities so that health care professionals will be better equipped to fulfill their important role in preventing, recognizing, and responding to commercial sexual exploitation and sex trafficking among the youth in their care.

HOW THIS GUIDE IS ORGANIZED

Following this introduction, Section 2 provides definitions of relevant terms, a set of guiding principles, a summary of what is known about the extent of the problem, and an overview of risk factors and consequences.

Section 3 reviews barriers to the ability of health care professionals to identify victims and survivors of these crimes, as well as some promising opportunities for overcoming these barriers.

Section 4 describes some ways in which health care professionals are responding to these crimes. It also summarizes multisector, collaborative strategies in which the health care sector plays a role.

Finally, Section 5 presents strategies for making progress in identifying, preventing, and responding to these crimes, based on the recommendations offered in the IOM/NRC report.

2   The Problem

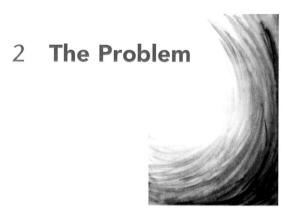

"Commercial sexual exploitation and sex trafficking
of minors should be understood as acts of abuse and
violence against children and adolescents."

This chapter first defines terms relevant to the problem of commercial
sexual exploitation and sex trafficking of minors in the United States. It
then presents a set of guiding principles that should inform any efforts
to address the problem. Next is a brief discussion of what is known about the
extent of the problem. The final section summarizes the current understanding of risk factors and consequences. One of the messages that emerges from
this discussion is that, while the gravity of the problem is clear, critical gaps
in the knowledge base for understanding and addressing it need to be filled.

THE DEFINITION ISSUE

The language used to describe aspects of commercial sexual exploitation
and sex trafficking crimes and their victims and survivors—a collection of
terms derived from the range of agencies, sectors, and individuals working
to prevent and address these crimes—varies considerably. Some terms are
diagnostic and scientific (e.g., *screening* and *medical forensic exam*). Others
are legal terms (e.g., *trafficking, offender, perpetrator*). Some terms are used
frequently in popular culture (e.g., *pimp, john, child prostitute*). Still others
are focused on the experiences of exploited children (e.g., *victim, survivor,*

modern-day slavery). The result is the absence of a shared language regarding commercial sexual exploitation and sex trafficking of minors.

The implications of this absence of a common language can be significant. For example, a child or adolescent victim identified as a prostitute may be treated as a criminal and detained, whereas the same youth identified as a victim of commercial sexual exploitation will be referred for a range of health and protective services. Box 1 provides the definition used in the IOM/NRC report for the commercial sexual exploitation and sex trafficking of minors. Box 2 presents the report's definitions for some of the more common terms related to these crimes.

Commercial sexual exploitation and *sex trafficking* of minors are distinct but overlapping terms. Indeed, disentangling commercial sexual exploitation from sex trafficking is impossible in many instances. Two points are particularly important for readers of this guide. First, programs designed for victims and survivors will need to account for a range of experiences and needs among those being served. Second, as reflected in the guiding principles presented in the next section, it is crucial to recognize and understand commercial sexual exploitation and sex trafficking of minors as part of a broader pattern of child abuse (as illustrated by Figure 1).

BOX 1
Definition of Commercial Sexual Exploitation
and Sex Trafficking of Minors

Commercial sexual exploitation and *sex trafficking of minors* encompass a range of crimes of a sexual nature committed against children and adolescents, including

- recruiting, enticing, harboring, transporting, providing, obtaining, and/or maintaining (acts that constitute trafficking) a minor for the purpose of sexual exploitation;
- exploiting a minor through prostitution;
- exploiting a minor through survival sex (exchanging sex/sexual acts for money or something of value, such as shelter, food, or drugs);
- using a minor in pornography;
- exploiting a minor through sex tourism, mail order bride trade, and early marriage; and
- exploiting a minor by having her/him perform in sexual venues (e.g., peep shows or strip clubs).

BOX 2
Definitions of Other Key Terms

Minors—Refers to individuals under age 18.

Prostituted child—Used instead of *child prostitute, juvenile prostitute,* and *adolescent prostitute*, which suggest that prostituted children are willing participants in an illegal activity. As stated in the guiding principles in the text below, these young people should be recognized as victims, not criminals.

Traffickers, exploiters, and pimps—Used to describe individuals who exploit children sexually for financial or other gain. In today's slang, pimp is often used to describe something as positive or glamorous. Therefore, the IOM/NRC report instead uses the terms trafficker and exploiter to describe individuals who sell children and adolescents for sex. It is also important to note that traffickers and exploiters come in many forms; they may be family members, intimate partners, or friends, as well as strangers.

Victims and survivors—Refers to minors who are commercially sexually exploited or trafficked for sexual purposes. The terms are not mutually exclusive, but can be applied to the same individual at different points along a continuum. The term *victim* indicates that a crime has occurred and that assistance is needed. Being able to identify an individual as a victim, even temporarily, can help activate responses—including direct services and legal protections—for an individual. The term *survivor* is also used because it can have therapeutic value, and the label *victim* may be counterproductive at times.

GUIDING PRINCIPLES

"Minors who are commercially sexually exploited or trafficked for sexual purposes should not be considered criminals."

The IOM/NRC report offers the following guiding principles as an essential foundation for understanding and responding to commercial sexual exploitation and sex trafficking of minors:

- Commercial sexual exploitation and sex trafficking of minors should be understood as acts of abuse and violence against children and adolescents.
- Minors who are commercially sexually exploited or trafficked for sexual purposes should not be considered criminals.
- Identification of victims and survivors and any intervention, above all, should do no further harm to any child or adolescent.

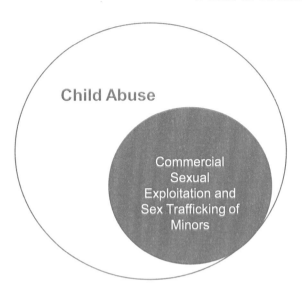

FIGURE 1 Commercial sexual exploitation and sex trafficking of minors are forms of child abuse.
NOTE: This diagram is for illustrative purposes only; it does not indicate or imply percentages.

EXTENT OF THE PROBLEM

> "Despite the current imperfect estimates, commercial sexual exploitation and sex trafficking of minors in the United States clearly are problems of grave concern."

Despite the gravity of commercial sexual exploitation and sex trafficking of minors in the United States, these crimes currently are not well understood or adequately addressed. Many factors contribute to this lack of understanding. For example:

- Commercial sexual exploitation and sex trafficking of minors in the United States may be overlooked and underreported because they frequently occur at the margins of society and behind closed doors. Their victims are often vulnerable to exploitation. They include children who are, or have been, neglected or abused; those in foster care or juvenile detention; and those who are homeless, runaways (i.e., children who leave home without permission), or so-called thrownaways (i.e., children and adolescents who are asked or told to leave home). Thus, children and adolescents affected by commercial sexual exploitation and sex trafficking can be difficult to reach.

- The absence of specific policies and protocols related to commercial sexual exploitation and sex trafficking of minors, coupled with a lack of specialized training, makes it difficult to identify—and thus count—victims and survivors of these crimes.
- Victims and survivors may be distrustful of law enforcement, may not view themselves as "victims," or may be too traumatized to report or disclose the crimes committed against them.
- Most states continue to arrest commercially exploited children and adolescents as criminals instead of treating them as victims, and health care professionals and educators have not widely adopted screening for commercial sexual exploitation and sex trafficking of minors. A lack of awareness among those who routinely interact with victims and survivors ensures that these crimes are not identified and properly addressed.

As a result of these factors, the true scope of commercial sexual exploitation and sex trafficking of minors within the United States is difficult to quantify, and estimates of the incidence and prevalence of commercial sexual exploitation and sex trafficking of minors in the United States are scarce. Further, there is little to no consensus on the value of existing estimates. This lack of consensus is not unusual and indeed is the case for estimates of other crimes as well (e.g., rape and intimate partner violence).

The IOM/NRC report maintains that, despite the current imperfect estimates, commercial sexual exploitation and sex trafficking of minors in the United States clearly are problems of grave concern. Therefore, the report's recommendations go beyond refining national estimates of commercial sexual exploitation and sex trafficking of minors in the United States to emphasize that unless additional resources become available existing resources should be focused on what can be done to assist the victims of these crimes.

RISK FACTORS

Risk factors for victims of commercial sexual exploitation and sex trafficking of minors have been identified at the individual, family, peer, neighborhood, and societal levels (see Figure 2).[1] Adding to this complexity, these risk factors, as well as corresponding protective factors, interact within and across levels.

Figure 2 highlights the complex and interconnected forces that contribute to commercial sexual exploitation and sex trafficking of minors. It should

---

[1]It should be noted that the evidence base for risk factors, as well as for consequences, is very limited. Therefore, the IOM/NRC report draws heavily on related literature (such as child maltreatment, sexual assault/rape, and trauma), as well as evidence gathered through workshops and site visits.

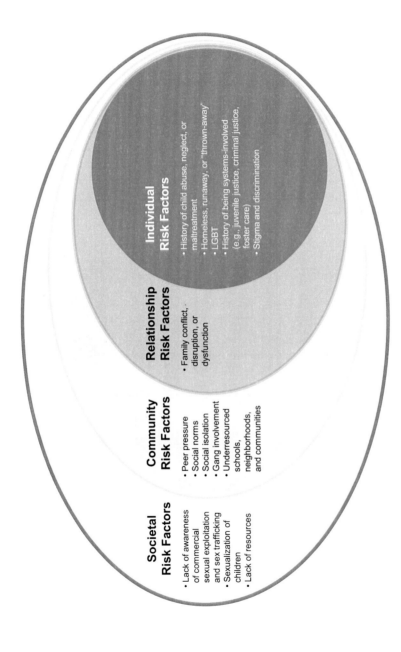

FIGURE 2 Possible risk factors for commercial sexual exploitation and sex trafficking of minors.
NOTE: LGBT = lesbian, gay, bisexual, or transgender.

be noted, however, that the factors shown are likely only a subset of the risk factors for these crimes. Moreover, these factors do not operate alone. For example, the presence of one or more risk factors would not result in the commercial sexual exploitation and sex trafficking of minors without the presence of an exploiter or trafficker. The factors depicted in Figure 2 may function independently of one another or in combination. In addition, risk factors in one sphere may trigger a cascade of effects or initiate pathways into or out of commercial sexual exploitation and sex trafficking.

Finally, the factors in Figure 2 also may be risks for other types of adverse youth outcomes. Therefore, their presence does not necessarily signal commercial sexual exploitation and sex trafficking of minors, but should be considered as part of a more comprehensive assessment to determine youth at risk of or involved in these crimes.

Box 3 summarizes findings from the IOM/NRC report that highlight the risk factors depicted in Figure 2.

CONSEQUENCES

"Overall, research suggests that victims and survivors of commercial sexual exploitation and sex trafficking face developmental, social, societal, and legal consequences that have both short- and long-term impacts on their health and well-being."

The available literature shows that child maltreatment, particularly child sexual abuse, has significant negative impacts on the physical health, mental health, and social functioning of victims in adulthood, and leads to increased health risk behaviors and mental health problems among adolescents. While studies focused on consequences for commercially sexually exploited children and adolescents are rare, the data based on child sexual abuse are useful given evidence that these problems are linked in some cases. Overall, research suggests that victims and survivors of commercial sexual exploitation and sex trafficking face developmental, social, societal, and legal consequences that have both short- and long-term impacts on their health and well-being.

BOX 3
Findings on Risk Factors

- Child maltreatment, particularly sexual abuse, is strongly associated with commercial sexual exploitation and sex trafficking of minors.
- Psychogenic factors, such as poor self-esteem, chronic depression, and external locus of control, in addition to low future orientation, may be risk factors for involvement in these crimes. This possible link is supported by the association between child maltreatment and these psychogenic factors.
- Off-schedule developmental phenomena, such as early pubertal maturation, early sexual participation, and early work initiation, have negative consequences for youth.
- While commercial sexual exploitation and sex trafficking can affect youth across the board, some groups are at higher risk, including those who lack stable housing (because of being homeless, runaways, or "thrown aways") and sexual and gender minority youth. In addition, some settings and situations—homelessness, foster care placement, and juvenile justice involvement—are particularly high risk under certain circumstances, providing opportunities for recruitment.
- Substance use/abuse is a risk factor for commercial sexual exploitation and sex trafficking of minors and also may perpetuate exploitation.
- The sexualization of children, particularly girls, in U.S. society and the perception that involvement in sex after puberty is consensual, contribute to the commercial sexual exploitation and sex trafficking of minors.
- Disability should be considered a vulnerability for involvement in these crimes given its association with child sexual abuse.
- Online and digital technologies are part of a complex social system that includes both risk factors (recruiting, grooming, and advertising victims) and protective factors (identifying, monitoring, and combating exploiters) for these crimes.
- Beyond child maltreatment, the experience of childhood adversity, such as growing up in a home with a family member with mental illness or substance abuse or having an incarcerated parent, may increase the risk for involvement in commercial sexual exploitation and sex trafficking of minors.
- Peer pressure and modeling can influence a youth's entry into (or avoidance of) commercial sexual exploitation.
- The neighborhood context—such as community norms about sexual behavior and what constitutes consent and coercion, and whether the community is characterized by poverty, crime, police corruption, adult prostitution, and high numbers of transient males—can increase the risk for involvement in these crimes.

3 Barriers to Identification of Victims and Survivors

"In contrast with intimate partner violence and child abuse, few health care settings have established screening practices, policies, and protocols related to commercial sexual exploitation and sex trafficking of minors."

Victims and survivors of commercial sexual exploitation and sex trafficking of minors may experience a variety of physical and mental health illnesses and injuries. Thus, they might be expected to present for treatment at some point during their exploitation. If each of these encounters is viewed as a potential opportunity to offer needed assistance, it would follow that health care professionals must be prepared to identify these youth and provide this assistance.

Yet a number of factors contribute to a failure to recognize and identify victims and survivors of these crimes among professionals not just in health care, but in all the various sectors that provide services to youth [9, 10, 11, 12]. Several of these factors are similar to those found to contribute to a failure to identify victims of child abuse and neglect [13]. These factors include, among others, a lack of understanding of commercial sexual exploitation and sex trafficking of minors (by both professionals and victims/survivors), a lack of disclosure by victims, potential and perceived complications related to mandated reporting, and a lack of policies and protocols related to these crimes to assist health care professionals in assessing and treating victims and survivors.

LACK OF UNDERSTANDING

Health care professionals need education and training to overcome a wide-spread lack of understanding of commercial sexual exploitation and sex trafficking of minors, which may prevent them from identifying and providing services to victims and survivors [14, 15, 16]. They need not only to be aware of the issue but also to have the knowledge and skills to identify and provide assistance to victims, survivors, and those at risk for exploitation, including reporting and referrals to other service providers. Among specific needs are training in confidentiality issues, identifying and gaining the trust of victims and survivors, collaboration and networking, outreach methods, medical and mental health issues, cultural and religious issues, and staffing challenges [17]. Yet a number of barriers to the training of health care professionals in these areas exist:

- **Stereotypes and misperceptions**—Two persistent stereotypes in particular may inhibit the identification of victims and survivors [4, 18, 19]: (1) the notion that the victims of these crimes are young, adolescent girls from foreign countries who are brought to the United States and coerced into prostitution [18], whereas in fact they include girls, boys, and transgender youth of different races/ethnicities and both domestic and international backgrounds; and (2) the tendency to label victims of these crimes who are minors as "child prostitutes" or to view them as being willingly engaged in criminal behavior [4, 19].
- **Lack of training opportunities**—Health care professionals may find it difficult to identify appropriate, well-designed training and education offered by individuals qualified to facilitate or provide it. Given that similar issues arise with domestic violence and child abuse and with commercial sexual exploitation and sex trafficking of minors, the current training of health care professionals in the former fields in medical and nursing schools, in residency, and during fellowships may provide an opportunity for improving training in the latter. Furthermore, many national health care organizations can help promote awareness through continuing medical education and sponsored training and meetings. Section 4 of this guide describes some current education and training programs that may meet this need but require further evaluation.
- **Funding constraints**—As in other areas of health care, limited funding is available with which to develop, provide, and evaluate training and curricula on commercial sexual exploitation and sex trafficking of minors for health care professionals [20, 21, 22].

- **Competing priorities**—Health care professionals are often over-burdened with mandatory training and education within their practice environments. It is important to note that simply adding another required educational topic, whether through in-person training or computer-based module, may not result in a more informed provider; education and training must be thoughtfully designed.

LACK OF DISCLOSURE

"These youth may not perceive themselves as victims or may believe that they are responsible for their exploitation."

An additional barrier to identifying victims and survivors is their lack of disclosure of being commercially sexually exploited or trafficked. This lack of disclosure may be due to a fear or distrust of professionals and the systems within which they operate [20, 23]. Victimized youth also may fear how their exploiter will respond to their disclosure [10, 12, 24, 25, 26]. These youth may be coached by their exploiter in how to answer questions from authority figures or health care professionals so as not to draw attention to their exploitation. Moreover, they may not perceive themselves as victims or may believe that they are responsible for their exploitation [4, 8, 10, 12]. Box 4 describes one potential approach to overcoming this barrier.

BOX 4
Overcoming the Barrier of Nondisclosure

Given the similar issues of nondisclosure encountered with victims of commercial sexual exploitation and sex trafficking and domestic violence, strategies used with victims of domestic violence may hold promise for overcoming lack of disclosure as a barrier to the identification of victims and survivors of commercial sexual exploitation and sex trafficking. Accordingly, some organizations seeking to help victims and survivors of these crimes have adapted a model screening protocol used for domestic violence. For example, Asian Health Services in Oakland, California, ensures that all patients are interviewed alone and uses interpreters of patients' native language to interview them instead of interviewing family members who may speak English [20].

POTENTIAL AND PERCEIVED COMPLICATIONS RELATED TO MANDATED REPORTING[1]

In all 50 states and the District of Columbia, health care professionals are mandated reporters, required to report all cases of suspected child abuse. In a significant number of states, however, mandatory reporting applies only when the suspected abuser is a family member or caregiver. Yet the perpetrators of commercial sexual exploitation and sex trafficking of minors are not always family members, and the victims are often not living at home. In those states, therefore, most commercial sexual exploitation and sex trafficking of minors does not fall within the mandatory reporting requirements.

Several states have passed legislation that makes commercial sexual exploitation and sex trafficking of minors by non-family members reportable forms of child abuse. Yet such mandated reporting could undermine health care professionals' willingness to screen for these crimes or respond to victims' voluntary disclosure [8, 27, 28, 29]. Clinicians may worry that reporting could make it more difficult to create trust with and obtain sensitive information from their patient. They also may worry that reporting may place victims at greater risk from their exploiters. Thus, to avoid the unintended consequences of being compelled to notify child protective services and/or other authorities, health care professionals may decide not to ask specific questions related to possible exploitation or trafficking [8, 27, 28, 29]. Clinicians' reservations about mandatory reporting are clear from published data showing that mandated reporting of child abuse and intimate partner violence makes health care professionals more reluctant to screen and intervene in these areas [30, 31, 32, 33, 34, 35]. Likewise, victims may not disclose their exploitation if they know or suspect that a health care professional will report it to the authorities.

LACK OF POLICIES AND PROTOCOLS

The kinds of established screening practices, policies, and protocols used for intimate partner violence and child abuse in health care settings do not exist for commercial sexual exploitation and sex trafficking of minors. Ideally, such policies and protocols should be evidence-based and evaluated for their effectiveness in assisting providers with identification, treatment, and referral for services.

---

[1]The IOM/NRC report [1, pp. 26-27] includes a detailed explanation of the complexities of mandatory reporting of commercial sexual exploitation and sex trafficking of minors in the United States in the context of the current practices of the legal, health care, and support service sectors. Available online: www.iom.edu/sextraffickingminors.

4 How Health Care Professionals Can Help

"Regardless of how they are identified, it is essential that health care professionals recognize and treat the myriad acute and chronic medical and mental health needs of minors who are victims or survivors of commercial sexual exploitation and sex trafficking."

The health care response to commercial sexual exploitation and sex trafficking of minors and research on the strengths and weaknesses of specific health care practices in this area are much less well developed than is the case for other health domains. However, the IOM/NRC report highlights a number of current practices and opportunities described by a variety of sources that show promise as ways of preventing commercial sexual exploitation and sex trafficking of minors and providing victims and survivors with the help they need. As emphasized in the IOM/NRC report, additional research is needed to evaluate these approaches for their efficacy in preventing or responding to these crimes (see the recommended strategies in Section 6).

MODELS OF CARE

Health care professionals lack evidence-based models to use in identifying and assisting victims of commercial sexual exploitation and sex trafficking of minors. However, the challenges they face in seeking to help these youth are similar to those encountered with intimate partner violence, child maltreatment, sexual assault services, and public health. Some agencies have therefore adapted models used in these fields to provide health care services to victims and survivors of commercial sexual exploitation and sex trafficking.

Intimate Partner Violence and Child Maltreatment

Many health care professionals have been trained to recognize victims of intimate partner violence and child abuse, and these skills could potentially be adapted for use in identifying victims of commercial sexual exploitation and sex trafficking of minors [29, 36]. Models of care for intimate partner violence and child maltreatment also may be applicable to commercial sexual exploitation and sex trafficking of minors given the similar risks, signs, symptoms, and emotional and social consequences shared by victims and survivors [20, 29, 36, 37, 38].

Sexual Assault Nurse Examiner (SANE)

Many victims of commercial sexual exploitation and sex trafficking have a history of childhood sexual assault and are sexually abused repeatedly as part of their exploitation. Therefore, intervention programs for victims and survivors of these crimes could potentially use the SANE program as a model.

SANE providers evaluate cases referred by their local jurisdiction using forensic interviews and forensic medical exams as part of a sexual assault investigation. The SANE examiners are already working in a system of care that is victim centered and collaborates with many of the same agencies likely to be encountered by a victim of commercial sexual exploitation or sex trafficking of minors (such as child protective services, law enforcement, and prosecutors). Thus, they could potentially provide the same kind of care to victims and survivors of these crimes [8, 29].

Integration of Services

Some agencies have integrated services and resources for victims and survivors of commercial sexual exploitation and sex trafficking into established child abuse and/or intimate partner violence programs. Two examples are described in Box 5.

Child Advocacy Centers and Sexual Assault Response Teams

Victims and survivors of commercial sexual exploitation and sex trafficking have multiple needs that cut across a number of different disciplines. Child advocacy centers (CACs) and sexual assault response teams (SARTs) both offer

BOX 5
Examples of Integrated Services

The Sexual Assault and Violence Intervention (SAVI) program at Mount Sinai Hospital in New York City has begun serving trafficking victims identified through the court system; referrals from other clients; and disclosure from a sexual assault evaluation, including such an evaluation in the health care setting [38]. These victims of commercial sexual exploitation and sex trafficking are provided free and confidential services, including case management, medical care, crisis shelter, legal assistance, and trauma therapy services, all of which are already provided to other sexual assault victims.

FOR MORE INFORMATION:

Sexual Assault and Violence Intervention Program.
http://www.mountsinai.org/patient-care/service-areas/community-medicine/areas-of-care/
sexual-assault-and-violence-intervention-program-savi

Asian Health Services in Oakland, California, has modified its screening tool for interpersonal violence for use in identifying victims of commercial sexual exploitation. It also has worked with those who deal with victims of interpersonal violence, including police investigators and health and mental health care professionals, to serve victims of commercial sexual exploitation as well as domestic violence victims [20].

FOR MORE INFORMATION:

Asian Health Services.
http://www.asianhealthservices.org

multidisciplinary services, and are therefore a potential model for identification, assessment, and management of victims and survivors of these crimes [29, 39]. The SAVI program described in Box 5 demonstrates the expansion of services provided to sexual assault victims by a SART center to include victims of these crimes. This approach may offer important advantages, particularly in those jurisdictions that lack specialized services for victims and survivors of commercial sexual exploitations and sex trafficking. At the same time, however, care must be taken to ensure that the services thus provided meet the special needs of these youth, which may exceed or differ from those of other youth served by CACs and SARTs.

Public Health

Commercial sexual exploitation and sex trafficking of minors are associated with several public health issues of concern to local communities, including domestic violence, child abuse and neglect, HIV and other sexually transmitted infections, unwanted pregnancies, basic unmet primary preventive health care needs among adolescents (e.g., immunizations, tuberculosis screening), drug and alcohol abuse and addiction, and numerous other often unmet medical and mental health needs [8, 40, 41]. Accordingly, some health care professionals and local communities have developed integrated programs to prevent and respond to these crimes through a public health model of care.

Asian Health Services in Oakland, California, for example, developed several such programs. These programs focus community efforts on (1) early primary prevention (e.g., education on healthy relationships for the younger adolescent population); (2) secondary prevention (identification of those at high risk for commercial sexual exploitation and sex trafficking and their referral to local service provider Banteay Srei [42], which provides resources to prevent them from becoming victims); and (3) tertiary prevention (e.g., a program to help those identified as victims and provide services to assist them in transitioning out of their victimization) [20]. Others have described a public health model for basing primary, secondary, and tertiary levels of prevention on the stage of trafficking of victims [10, 40].

Telehealth/Telemedicine

Telehealth has been used successfully to deliver care for sexually abused children in rural, underserved areas [43, 44], for adolescents and children needing psychiatric services [45, 46], and for victims of domestic violence and sexual assault in rural communities [47]. Similarly, health care professionals who may lack the resources for evaluation, referral, and/or assistance for victims and survivors of commercial sexual exploitation and sex trafficking within their own communities may be able to use telehealth to access those resources.

EDUCATION AND TRAINING OF HEALTH CARE PROFESSIONALS

As discussed in Section 3, a lack of training is a significant barrier to the ability of health care professionals to identify victims and survivors of commercial sexual exploitation and sex trafficking. To help overcome this barrier, a growing number of organizations providing services to victimized or at-risk youth are offering education and training programs for health care professionals [26, 48, 49]. However, the vast majority of training developed for health care professionals focuses on the broader topic of human trafficking, and although content on commercial sexual exploitation and sex trafficking of minors may be included, programs specific to these issues are lacking.

Programs identified in the IOM/NRC report were designed to help health care professionals recognize the signs and symptoms of commercial sexual exploitation and sex trafficking, provide tools for screening, and highlight reporting requirements and how/when to refer victims and survivors for additional services [20, 21, 26, 27, 48, 49, 50, 51, 52]. Three examples are described in Box 6.

BOX 6
Examples of Education and Training Programs

The Houston Rescue and Restore Coalition (HRRC) is a nonprofit organization in Houston, Texas, focused on raising awareness of human trafficking. In collaboration with the University of Texas School of Public Health, it developed a curriculum titled "Health Professionals and Human Trafficking: Look Beneath the Surface, H.E.A.R.[a] Your Patient" for front-line health care professionals and health care organizations [53]. The intent is to provide health care professionals with not only the information and knowledge but also the skills necessary to identify and refer trafficking victims.

FOR MORE INFORMATION:

Houston Rescue and Restore Coalition.
http://www.houstonrr.org

Children's Health Care of Atlanta, along with the Georgia Governor's Office for Children and Families, developed and provided training for medical professionals via a webinar/computer-based training series. The five-session series provides an overview of commercial sexual exploitation of minors, the medical evaluation of suspected victims, extended medical history, special related topics, and a victim/survivor-centered approach to working with these youth [51].

FOR MORE INFORMATION:

Children's Health Care of Atlanta. Child Sex Trafficking Webinar Series.
http://www.choa.org/csecwebinars

Polaris Project offers free, online training and webinars that provide education and training on various topics related to human trafficking and sex trafficking in particular.

FOR MORE INFORMATION:

Polaris Project. Online Training.
http://www.polarisproject.org/what-we-do/national-human-trafficking-hotline/access-training/online-training

---

[a] H.E.A.R. is an acronym for H: Human Trafficking and Health Professionals, E: Examine History, Examine Body, Examine Emotion, A: Ask specific questions, and R: Review options, Refer, Report.

TOOLS FOR IDENTIFICATION OF VICTIMS

Box 7 describes a variety of tools, instruments, and lists of questions designed to assist health care professionals in identifying victims and survivors of commercial sexual exploitation and sex trafficking. Again, none of these tools have as yet been evaluated for their ability to correctly identify these youth.

The agencies and providers that developed these screening tools emphasize the need for health care professionals to be aware of the unique experiences of victims and survivors of these crimes (such as repeat and/or chronic sexual victimization, potential stigma and shame associated with victimization, and possible negative interactions with authority figures and support systems). Specifically, it is recommended that the tools be used by

---

BOX 7
Examples of Tools for Identifying Victims and Survivors
of Commercial Sexual Exploitation and Sex Trafficking

The following tools have been developed to assist health care professionals in identifying victims and survivors of commercial sexual exploitation and sex trafficking:

- Rapid Screening Tool for Child Trafficking and Comprehensive Screening and Safety Tool for Child Trafficking: Two screening tools developed by the International Organization for Adolescents for use as a guide in identifying minors that are potentially being trafficked [54].
- Commercial Sexually Exploited Children (CSEC) Screening Procedure Guideline: A screening tool developed and used by health care professionals at Asian Health Services in Oakland, California, that is used with patients aged 11-18 exhibiting high risk factors for sexual exploitation [55].
- Rescue and Restore: A screening tool developed by the U.S. Department of Health and Human Services and used by health care professionals, social workers, and law enforcement to determine potential victims of human trafficking [56].
- Comprehensive Human Trafficking Assessment: A screening tool developed by the National Human Trafficking Resource Center and adapted by Polaris Project and its partners for assessing potential signs of a client's having been a victim of human trafficking [57].
- Home, Education/employment, peer group Activities, Drugs, Sexuality, Suicide/depression (HEADSS) [58]: A screening tool developed for assessing an adolescent's psychosocial development. Mount Sinai Adolescent Health Center has adopted HEADSS, integrating specific questions into its regular assessment to screen for the potential of commercial sexual exploitation among patients seen in the clinic [49].

providers who are trained in or understand the nature of the trauma these particular victims and survivors suffer. The emphasis is on the importance of being trauma-aware when screening for commercial sexual exploitation and working with identified victims and survivors [8, 29, 12, 59, 60, 61].

HEALTH CARE OF VICTIMS AND SURVIVORS: MANAGEMENT AND TREATMENT

Regardless of how they are identified, minors who are victims or survivors of commercial sexual exploitation and sex trafficking have myriad acute and chronic physical and mental health needs. It is essential that health care professionals recognize and respond to these complex needs, which include not only basic primary preventive care services but also specialized services such as substance abuse treatment, chronic illness management (e.g., HIV, hepatitis B/C, diabetes, asthma, depression, anxiety), ongoing assessment and refilling of essential prescriptions, and overall and specific dental care [27, 62, 63]. Moreover, health care professionals who identify victims and survivors of commercial sexual exploitation and sex trafficking of minors likely will need to refer patients to other specialists, including mental health professionals and local nongovernmental organizations/agencies that can meet the specific mental health needs of these youth. They should be active in the development and implementation of the kinds of multisector approaches discussed below.

MULTISECTOR AND INTERAGENCY EFFORTS

Each of the sectors involved in responding to commercial sexual exploitation and sex trafficking of minors—victim and support services, health care, education, the legal sector, and the commercial sector—has specific roles to play. However, an adequate response to these crimes requires collaboration and coordination among all of these sectors, as well as at all levels—federal, state, and local. Yet the efforts of individuals, groups, and organizations in different sectors and with different areas of expertise tend to be disconnected. The IOM/NRC report highlights a number of examples of initiatives that have overcome this barrier to a comprehensive response.

Multisector and interagency efforts to address commercial sexual exploitation and sex trafficking of minors at the federal level include task forces and other partnerships, such as those mandated by the 2013 reauthorization of the Trafficking Victims Protection Act [54, 64, 65, 66].

FOR MORE INFORMATION:

BJA (Bureau of Justice Assistance). 2013. Anti-Human Trafficking Task Force Initiative.
https://www.bja.gov/ProgramDetails.aspx?Program_ID=51

Cook County Human Trafficking Task Force.
http://www.cookcountytaskforce.org

OVC (Office for Victims of Crime). 2013. OVC-Funded Grantee Programs to Help Victims of Trafficking.
http://www.ojp.gov/ovc/grants/traffickingmatrix.html

OVC and BJA. 2011. Anti-Human Trafficking Task Force Strategy and Operations E-guide.
https://www.ovcttac.gov/TaskForceGuide/EGuide/Default.aspx

OVC and BJA. 2013. Enhanced Collaborative Model to Combat Human Trafficking FY 2013 Competitive Grant Announcement.
https://www.bja.gov/Funding/13HumanTraffickingSol.pdf

President's Interagency Task Force to Monitor and Combat Trafficking in Persons. 2013. Federal Strategic Action Plan on Services for Victims of Human Trafficking in the United States 2013-2017.
http://ideascale.com//userimages/accounts/91/912839/Victim-Services-SAP-2013-04-09-Public-Comment-B.pdf

U.S. Attorney's Office for the District of Columbia. 2013. The D.C. Human Trafficking Task Force.
http://www.justice.gov/usao/dc/programs/cp/human_trafficking.html

U.S. Department of State. 2012. Annual Meeting of the President's Interagency Task Force to Monitor and Combat Trafficking in Persons.
http://www.state.gov/j/tip/rls/reports/pitf

Examples of state and local efforts include the following:

- **Washington State**—Washington state's Model Protocol for Commercially Sexually Exploited Children for responding to cases of commercial sexual exploitation and sex trafficking of minors is focused on fostering collaboration and coordination among agencies, improving identification of these crimes, providing services to victims and survivors, holding exploiters accountable, and working toward ending these crimes in the state [67]. The protocol calls for use of a victim-centered approach by law enforcement, the courts, victim advocacy organizations, youth service agencies, and other youth-serving professionals to ensure that victims of these crimes are treated as such rather than as criminals. The protocol encourages multisector collaboration through state, regional, and local efforts. For example, it calls for the use of multidisciplinary teams to provide immediate consultation on cases of commercial sexual exploitation and sex trafficking of minors as they arise and to participate in meetings to share information and collaborate in the management of each ongoing case.

FOR MORE INFORMATION:

Washington State's Model Protocol for Commercially Sexually Exploited Children.
http://www.ccyj.org/Project%20Respect%20protocol.pdf

- **Multnomah County, Oregon**—In 2008, Multnomah County initiated a coordinated multisector response to commercial sexual exploitation and sex trafficking of minors. Specific work groups focus on legislation, assistance for victims and survivors, law enforcement practices (e.g., arrests, investigation, and prosecution of exploiters and traffickers), and physical and mental health care. Steering committee members include law enforcement; the district attorney's office; the Departments of Health, Community Justice, and Human Services; survivors; and nongovernmental service providers. Several strategies are used to ensure collaboration across agencies and among various systems. For example, the county created a special unit within the state child welfare agency for victims and survivors of these crimes [68, 69].

FOR MORE INFORMATION:

Multnomah County Community Response to Commercial Sexual Exploitation of Children.
https://multco.us/csec

- **Suffolk County, Massachusetts**—In Suffolk County, more than 35 public and private agencies participate in the Support to End Exploitation Now (SEEN) Coalition. SEEN's multisector, coordinated approach to identifying and serving high-risk and sexually exploited

minors includes three components: (1) cross-system collaboration, (2) a trauma-informed continuum of care (see Section 4), and
(3) training for professionals who work with children and adolescents. To facilitate collaboration and communication among coalition members, SEEN established formal relationships and protocols,
including a steering committee and advisory group, multidisciplinary
teams of professionals, and a case coordinator who serves as the
central point of contact for all reported victims of commercial sexual
exploitation and sex trafficking [70].

FOR MORE INFORMATION:

Support to End Exploitation Now (SEEN) Coalition.
http://www.suffolkcac.org/programs/seen

- **Alameda County, California**—H.E.A.T. (Human Exploitation and
Trafficking) Watch is a multidisciplinary, multisystem program that
brings together individuals and agencies from law enforcement,
health care, advocacy, victim and support services, the courts, probation agencies, the commercial sector, and the community to (1) ensure the safety of victims and survivors and (2) pursue accountability
for exploiters and traffickers. Strategies employed by H.E.A.T. Watch
include, among others, stimulating community engagement, coordinating training and information sharing, and coordinating the delivery of victim and support services. The program uses a multisector
approach to coordinate the delivery of support services. For example,
multidisciplinary case review (modeled on the multidisciplinary team
approach) is used to create emergency and long-term safety plans.
Referrals for case review are made by law enforcement, prosecutors,
probation officials, and social service organizations that have come
into contact with these youth. This approach enables members of
the multidisciplinary team to share confidential information with
agencies that can assist youth in need of services and support.

FOR MORE INFORMATION:

*Alameda County District Attorney's Office. 2012. H.E.A.T. Watch
Program Blueprint.*
http://www.heat-watch.org/heat_watch

5 Recommended Strategies

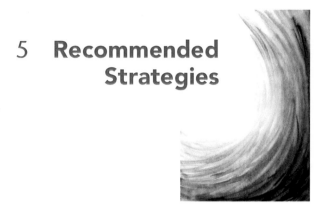

The IOM/NRC report concludes with a series of recommendations for making progress toward preventing and responding to commercial sexual exploitation and sex trafficking of minors in the United States. The priorities for progress articulated in the report's recommendations are summarized in this section.

INCREASE AWARENESS AND UNDERSTANDING

As discussed in prior sections, a lack of training among professionals who interact with children and adolescents—especially those who are vulnerable—is a barrier to timely and appropriate action to assist victims and survivors of commercial sexual exploitation and sex trafficking and prevent these crimes among youth at risk. These professionals are often dismayed to learn that they have missed opportunities to help these youth, and want to know more about how to identify and assist them.

Training

Training for professionals and others who interact with young people needs to target and reach a range of audiences in a variety of settings (e.g., urban

**RECOMMENDATION TO INCREASE
AWARENESS AND UNDERSTANDING**

Develop, implement, and evaluate:

- training for professionals and others who routinely interact with children and adolescents,
- public awareness campaigns, and
- specific strategies for children and adolescents.

and rural; tribal lands, territories, and states). Relevant sectors (e.g., health care, law enforcement, victim and support services) should participate in the development, implementation, and evaluation of training activities that use evidence-based methods. Further, each sector should be consulted to determine the best methods for that sector, given that needs may vary, for example, between law enforcement personnel and health care professionals.

Public Awareness Campaigns

A lack of public awareness is a significant barrier to preventing, identifying, and responding to commercial sexual exploitation and sex trafficking of minors in the United States. To address this gap, existing public awareness initiatives could be expanded to encompass these crimes.

Strategies for Awareness Among Children and Adolescents

Child and adolescent victims and survivors of commercial sexual exploitation and sex trafficking may not view themselves as victims, and youth who are at risk for this kind of exploitation may not recognize their individual risk. Therefore, special efforts are needed to increase the awareness of children and adolescents to help them avoid becoming victims and to help victims and survivors obtain the assistance they need.

STRENGTHEN THE LAW'S RESPONSE

"Individuals who sexually exploit children and adolescents have largely escaped accountability."

A small but growing number of states have enacted laws—sometimes referred to as "safe harbor" laws—designed to redirect young victims of commercial sexual exploitation and sex trafficking from the criminal or juvenile justice system to child welfare or other agencies to receive supportive services. While recognizing that additional time and research are needed to assess the effectiveness of specific state laws, the IOM/NRC report recommends that the core principle underlying these safe harbor laws—that children and adolescents who are survivors of sexual exploitation and sex trafficking must be treated as victims, not criminals—should be advanced without delay.

In addition, despite laws in every state that enable the prosecution of individuals who purchase sex with a minor, function as exploiters and traffickers, or otherwise sexually exploit children and adolescents, and despite the hard work of prosecutors and law enforcement in many jurisdictions, individuals who sexually exploit children and adolescents have largely escaped accountability.

RECOMMENDATIONS TO STRENGTHEN THE LAW'S RESPONSE

Develop laws and policies that **redirect** young victims and survivors of commercial sexual exploitation and sex trafficking from arrest and prosecution to systems, agencies, and services that are equipped to meet their needs. *Such laws should apply to all children and adolescents under age 18.*

Review, strengthen, and implement laws that hold exploiters, traffickers, and solicitors **accountable** for their role in commercial sexual exploitation and sex trafficking of minors. *These laws should include a particular emphasis on deterring demand.*

STRENGTHEN RESEARCH ON PREVENTION AND INTERVENTION

As noted previously, the evidence base on strategies and approaches for preventing and responding to commercial sexual exploitation and sex trafficking of minors in the United States is extremely limited.

RECOMMENDATION TO STRENGTHEN RESEARCH ON PREVENTION AND INTERVENTION

Implement a national research agenda focused on:

- advancing knowledge and understanding;
- developing effective interventions; and
- evaluating the effectiveness of prevention and intervention laws, policies, and programs.

SUPPORT COLLABORATION

As discussed in Section 3, collaborative, coordinated approaches that bring together resources from multiple sectors will be most effective in identifying victims and survivors and in meeting their challenging needs.

RECOMMENDATION TO SUPPORT COLLABORATION AND COORDINATION

Develop **guidelines** on and provide **technical assistance** to support multisector collaboration and coordination.

SUPPORT INFORMATION SHARING

"The difficulty of locating services and programs available to victims is a very real obstacle for children and adolescents seeking to access services and for professionals and caregivers trying to help them."

One of the most significant barriers to preventing, identifying, and responding to commercial sexual exploitation and sex trafficking of minors is a lack of reliable, timely information. A number of organizations maintain lists of services available to child and adolescent victims of commercial sexual exploitation and sex trafficking. However, there is no exhaustive list of national-, state-, local-, and tribal-level resources for victim and support services. The difficulty of locating services and programs available to victims is a very real obstacle for children and adolescents seeking to access services and for professionals and caregivers trying to help them.

RECOMMENDATION TO SUPPORT INFORMATION SHARING

Create and maintain a digital information-sharing platform to deliver **reliable, real-time information** on how to prevent, identify, and respond to commercial sexual exploitation and sex trafficking of minors in the United States.

FINAL THOUGHTS

Efforts to prevent, identify, and respond to commercial sexual exploitation and sex trafficking of minors in the United States are in the same developmental stage that efforts to deal with physical and sexual abuse of children were in during the 1970s, when a handful of multidisciplinary approaches for addressing those problems were emerging around the country. Approaches to domestic and interpersonal violence were at a similar stage in the early 1980s. The nation today has a real opportunity to build on lessons from those earlier efforts, as well as current noteworthy practices, to address the problem of commercial sexual exploitation and sex trafficking of minors, and the health care sector has a crucial role to play in achieving this goal. The children and adolescents who are at risk and are victims and survivors of these crimes cannot wait. The human cost of the status quo is simply unacceptable.

References

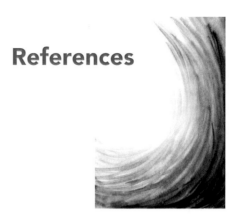

1. IOM (Institute of Medicine) and NRC (National Research Council). 2013. *Confronting commercial sexual exploitation and sex trafficking of minors in the United States.* Washington, DC: The National Academies Press.
2. Cohen, S. A. 2005. Ominous convergence: Sex trafficking, prostitution and international family planning. *The Guttmacher Report on Public Policy* 8(1):12-14.
3. Clawson, H. J., N. M. Dutch, A. Solomon, and L. Goldblatt Grace. 2009. *Human trafficking into and within the United States: A review of the literature.* Washington, DC: U.S. Department of Health and Human Services, Office of the Assistant Secretary for Planning and Evaluation.
4. Clawson, H. J., N. M. Dutch, A. Solomon, and L. Goldblatt Grace. 2009. *Study of HHS programs serving human trafficking victims.* Washington, DC: U.S. Department of Health and Human Services, Office of the Assistant Secretary for Planning and Evaluation.
5. Irazola, S., E. Williamson, C. Chen, A. Garrett, and H. J. Clawson. 2008. *Trafficking of U.S. citizens and legal permanent residents: The forgotten victims and survivors.* Washington, DC: ICF International.
6. Logan, T. K., R. Walker, and G. Hunt. 2009. Understanding human trafficking in the United States. *Trauma, Violence, and Abuse* 10(1):3-30.
7. Macy, R. J., and L. M. Graham. 2012. Identifying domestic and international sex-trafficking victims during human service provision. *Trauma Violence and Abuse* 13(2):59-76.
8. Williamson, E., N. M. Dutch, and H. J. Clawson. 2009. *National symposium on the health needs of human trafficking victims: Post-symposium brief.* Washington, DC: U.S. Department of Health and Human Services, Office of the Assistant Secretary for Planning and Evaluation.
9. Clawson, H. J., and N. Dutch. 2008. *Case management and the victim of human trafficking: A critical service for client success.* Washington, DC: U.S. Department of Health and Human Services, Office of the Assistant Secretary for Planning and Evaluation.

10. Crane, P. A., and M. Moreno. 2011. Human trafficking: What is the role of the health care provider? *Journal of Applied Research on Children: Informing Policy for Children at Risk* 2(1).

11. Lillywhite, R., and P. Skidmore. 2006. Boys are not sexually exploited?: A challenge to practitioners. *Child Abuse Review* 15(5):351-361.

12. Smith, L., S. H. Vardaman, and M. A. Snow. 2009. *The national report on domestic minor sex trafficking: America's prostituted children.* Vancouver, WA: Shared Hope International.

13. IOM (Institute of Medicine). 2002. *Confronting chronic neglect: The education and training of health professionals on family violence.* Washington, DC: National Academy Press.

14. Clawson, H. J., and L. Goldblatt Grace. 2007. *Finding a path to recovery: Residential facilities for minor victims of domestic sex trafficking.* Washington, DC: U.S. Department of Health and Human Services, Office of the Assistant Secretary for Planning and Evaluation.

15. Fong, R., and J. Berger Cardoso. 2010. Child human trafficking victims: Challenges for the child welfare system. *Evaluation and Program Planning* 33(3):311-316.

16. Okech, D., W. Morreau, and K. Benson. 2011. Human trafficking: Improving victim identification and service provision. *International Social Work* 55(4):488-503.

17. Clawson, H. J., K. Small, E. S. Go, and B. W. Myles. 2013. *Needs assessment for service providers and trafficking victims.* Fairfax, VA: Caliber Associates, Inc.

18. Clawson, H. J., and N. Dutch. 2008. *Identifying victims of human trafficking: Inherent challenges and promising strategies from the field.* Washington, DC: U.S. Department of Health and Human Services, Office of the Assistant Secretary for Planning and Evaluation.

19. Farley, M., and V. Kelly. 2000. Prostitution: A critical review of the medical and social sciences literature. *Women and Criminal Justice* 11(4):29-64.

20. Chang, K. S. G. 2012. Workshop presentation to the Committee on the Commercial Sexual Exploitation and Sex Trafficking of Minors in the United States, on the Asian Health Services, May 9, 2012, San Francisco, CA.

21. Goldblatt Grace, L., M. Starck, J. Potenza, P. A. Kenney, and A. H. Sheetz. 2012. Commercial sexual exploitation of children and the school nurse. *The Journal of School Nursing* 28(6):410-417.

22. Siffermann, W. P. 2012. Site visit presentation to the Committee on the Commercial Sexual Exploitation and Sex Trafficking of Minors in the United States, on the San Francisco Juvenile Probation Department, May 11, 2012, San Francisco, CA.

23. Nguyen, S. 2012. Workshop presentation to the Committee on the Commercial Sexual Exploitation and Sex Trafficking of Minors in the United States, on the Oakland High School Wellness Center, May 9, 2012, San Francisco, CA.

24. Holzman, J. 2012. Presentation to the Committee on the Commercial Sexual Exploitation and Sex Trafficking of Minors in the United States, on the Girls Educational and Mentoring Services (GEMS) services and programs, September 12, 2012, New York.

25. Miller, E., M. R. Decker, J. G. Silverman, and A. Raj. 2007. Migration, sexual exploitation, and women's health: A case report from a community health center. *Violence Against Women* 13(5):486-497.

26. Ring, M. 2012. Workshop presentation to the Committee on the Commercial Sexual Exploitation and Sex Trafficking of Minors in the United States, on the Standing Against Global Exploitation, May 12, 2012, San Francisco, CA.

27. Dovydaitis, T. 2009. Human trafficking: The role of the health care provider. *Journal of Midwifery and Women's Health* 55(5):462-467.

28. Durborow, N., K. C. Lizdas, A. O'Flaherty, and A. Marjavi. 2010. *Compendium of state statutes and policies on domestic violence and health care.* San Francisco, CA: Family Violence Prevention Fund.

29. Williamson, E., N. M. Dutch, and H. J. Clawson. 2010. *Medical treatment of victims of sexual assault and domestic violence and its applicability to victims of human trafficking.* Washington, DC: U.S. Department of Health and Human Services, Office of the Assistant Secretary for Planning and Evaluation.

30. Davidov, D. M., M. R. Nadorff, S. M. Jack, J. H. Coben, and NFP IVP Research Team. 2012. Nurse home visitors' perspectives of mandatory reporting of children's exposure to intimate partner violence to child protection agencies. *Public Health Nursing* 29(5):412-423.

31. Flaherty, E. G., and R. Sege. 2005. Barriers to physician identification and reporting of child abuse. *Pediatric Annals* 34(5):349-356.

32. Flaherty, E. G., R. Sege, L. L. Price, K. K. Christoffel, D. P. Norton, and K. G. O'Connor. 2006. Pediatrician characteristics associated with child abuse identification and reporting: Results from a national survey of pediatricians. *Child Maltreatment* 11(4):361-369.

33. Flaherty, E. G., R. D. Sege, J. Griffith, L. L. Price, R. Wasserman, E. Slora, N. Dhepyasuwan, D. Harris, D. Norton, M. L. Angelilli, D. Abney, and H. J. Binns. 2008. From suspicion of physical child abuse to reporting: Primary care clinician decision-making. *Pediatrics* 122(3):611-619.

34. Vulliamy, A. P., and R. Sullivan. 2000. Reporting child abuse: Pediatricians' experiences with the child protection system. *Child Abuse and Neglect* 24(11):1461-1470.

35. Warner, J. E., and D. J. Hansen. 1994. The identification and reporting of physical abuse by physicians: A review and implications for research. *Child Abuse and Neglect* 18(1):11-25.

36. Pearce, J. 2006. Who needs to be involved in safeguarding sexually exploited young people? *Child Abuse Review* 15(5):326-340.

37. Lalor, K., and R. McElvaney. 2010. Child sexual abuse, links to later sexual exploitation/ high-risk sexual behavior, and prevention/treatment programs. *Trauma, Violence, and Abuse* 11(4):159-177.

38. Latimer, D. 2012. Site visit presentation to the Committee on the Commercial Sexual Exploitation and Sex Trafficking of Minors in the United States, on the Mount Sinai Sexual Assault and Violence Intervention (SAVI) Program, September 12, 2012, New York.

39. Mitchell, K., D. Finkelhor, L. Jones, and J. Wolak. 2010. Growth and change in undercover online child exploitation investigations, 2000-2006. *Policing and Society* 20(4):416-431.

40. Zimmerman, C., M. Hossain, and C. Watts. 2011. Human trafficking and health: A conceptual model to inform policy, intervention and research. *Social Science and Medicine* 73(2):327-335.

41. Zimmerman, C., and C. Watts. 2007. Documenting the effects of trafficking in women. In *Public health and human rights: Evidence-based approaches,* edited by C. Breyer and H. F. Pizer. Baltimore, MD: The Johns Hopkins University Press.

42. Asian Health Services and Banteay Srei. 2012. *Programs.* http://banteaysrei.org (accessed April 16, 2013).

43. MacLeod, K. J., J. P. Marcin, C. Boyle, S. Miyamoto, R. J. Dimand, and K. K. Rogers. 2009. Using telemedicine to improve the care delivered to sexually abused children in rural, underserved hospitals. *Pediatrics* 123(1):223-228.

44. Thraen, I. M., L. Frasier, C. Cochella, J. Yaffe, and P. Goede. 2008. The use of telecam as a remote web-based application for child maltreatment assessment, peer review, and case documentation. *Child Maltreatment* 13(4):368-376.

45. Myers, K. M., J. M. Valentine, and S. M. Melzer. 2007. Feasibility, acceptability, and sustainability of telepsychiatry for children and adolescents. *Psychiatric Services* 58(11):1493-1496.

46. Myers, K. M., A. Vander Stoep, C. A. McCarty, J. B. Klein, N. B. Palmer, J. R. Geyer, and S. M. Melzer. 2010. Child and adolescent telepsychiatry: Variations in utilization, referral patterns and practice trends. *Journal of Telemedicine and Telecare* 16(3):128-133.

47. Hassija, C., and M. J. Gray. 2011. The effectiveness and feasibility of videoconferencing technology to provide evidence-based treatment to rural domestic violence and sexual assault populations. *Telemedicine and E-Health* 17(4):309-315.

48. Phillips, M. 2012. Workshop presentation to the Committee on the Commercial Sexual Exploitation and Sex Trafficking of Minors in the United States, on the Motivating, Inspiring, Supporting, and Serving Sexually Exploited Youth (MISSEY), May 9, 2012.

49. Steever, J. 2012. Site visit presentation to the Committee on the Commercial Sexual Exploitation and Sex Trafficking of Minors in the United States, on the Mount Sinai Adolescent Health Center, September 12, 2012, New York.

50. Goldblatt Grace, L. 2012. Site visit presentation to the Committee on the Commercial Sexual Exploitation and Sex Trafficking of Minors in the United States, on My Life, My Choice, March 23, 2012, Boston, MA.

51. Greenbaum, V. J. 2012. Workshop presentation to the Committee on Commercial Sexual Exploitation and Sex Trafficking of Minors in the United States, on the Children's Healthcare of Atlanta, May 9, 2012, San Francisco, CA.

52. Polenberg, M., and J. Westmacott. 2012. Site visit presentation to the Committee on Commercial Sexual Exploitation and Sex Trafficking of Minors in the United States, on the Safe Horizon services, September 12, 2012, New York.

53. Isaac, R., J. Solak, and A. P. Giardino. 2011. Health care providers' training needs related to human trafficking: Maximizing the opportunity to effectively screen and intervene. *Journal of Applied Research on Children: Informing Policy for Children at Risk* 2(1).

54. Walts, K. K., S. French, H. Moore, and S. Ashai. 2011. *Building child welfare response to child trafficking.* Chicago, IL: Loyola University Chicago, Center for the Human Rights of Children.

55. Asian Health Services and Banteay Srei. 2012. *Asian Health Services and Banteay Srei CSEC Screening Protocol.* http://www.asianhealthservices.org/docs/CSEC_Protocol.pdf (accessed April 11, 2013).

56. Administration for Children and Families, Office of Refugee Resettlement. 2012. *Rescue & Restore Campaign Tool Kits.* http://www.acf.hhs.gov/programs/orr/resource/rescue-restore-campaign-tool-kits (accessed April 11, 2013).

57. Polaris Project. 2012. *Tools for service providers and law enforcement.* http://www.polaris project.org/resources/tools-for-service-providers-and-law-enforcement (accessed April 10, 2013).

58. Goldenring, J., and E. Cohen. 1988. Getting into adolescents heads. *Contemporary Pediatrics* 5(7):75-80. 59.Clawson, H. J., A. Salomon, and L. Goldblatt Grace. 2008. *Treating the hidden wounds: Trauma treatment and mental health recovery for victims of human trafficking.* Washington, DC: U.S. Department of Health and Human Services, Office of the Assistant Secretary for Planning and Evaluation.

60. Lebloch, E. K., and S. King. 2006. Child sexual exploitation: A partnership response and model intervention. *Child Abuse Review* 15(5):362-372.

61. Hossain, M., C. Zimmerman, M. Abas, M. Light, and C. Watts. 2010. The relationship of trauma to mental disorders among trafficked and sexually exploited girls and women. *American Journal of Public Health* 100(12):2442-2449.

62. Sabella, D. 2011. The role of the nurse in combating human trafficking. *American Journal of Nursing* 111(2):28-37.

63. Zimmerman, C., M. Hossain, K. Yun, V. Gajdadziev, N. Guzun, M. Tchomarova, R. A. Ciarrocchi, A. Johansson, A. Kefurtova, and S. Scodanibbio. 2008. The health of traf-ficked women: A survey of women entering posttrafficking services in Europe. *American Journal of Public Health* 98(1):55-59.

64. Knowles-Wirsing, E. 2012. Workshop presentation to the Committee on the Commer-cial Sexual Exploitation and Sex Trafficking of Minors in the United States, on Salvation Army STOP-IT, July 11, 2012, Chicago, IL.

65. Greene, J. 2012. Site visit presentation to the Committee on the Commercial Sexual Exploitation and Sex Trafficking of Minors in the United States, on the Cook County State's Attorney's Office, Human Trafficking Task Force, July 11, 2012, Chicago, IL.

66. Nasser, M. 2012. Site visit presentation to the Committee on the Commercial Sexual Exploitation and Sex Trafficking of Minors in the United States, on the U.S. Attorney's Office, Northern District of Illinois, July 11, 2012, Chicago, IL.

67. Bridge, B. J., N. Oakley, L. Briner, and B. Graef. 2012. *Washington state model protocol for commercially sexually exploited children.* Seattle, WA: Center for Children and Youth Justice.

68. Baker, J., and E. Nelson. 2012. Workshop presentation to the Committee on the Com-mercial Sexual Exploitation and Sex Trafficking of Minors in the United States, on multi-disciplinary responses, May 9, 2012, San Francisco, CA.

69. Multnomah County. 2012. *Multnomah County: Community response to Commercial Sexual Exploitation of Children (CSEC).* Multnomah County, OR: Department of Com-munity Justice.

70. Piening, S., and T. Cross. 2012. *From "the life" to my life: Sexually exploited children reclaiming their futures Suffolk County Massachusetts' response to Commercial Sexual Ex-ploitation of Children (CSEC).* Boston, MA: Children's Advocacy Center of Suffolk County.